YOGA
for Stuttering

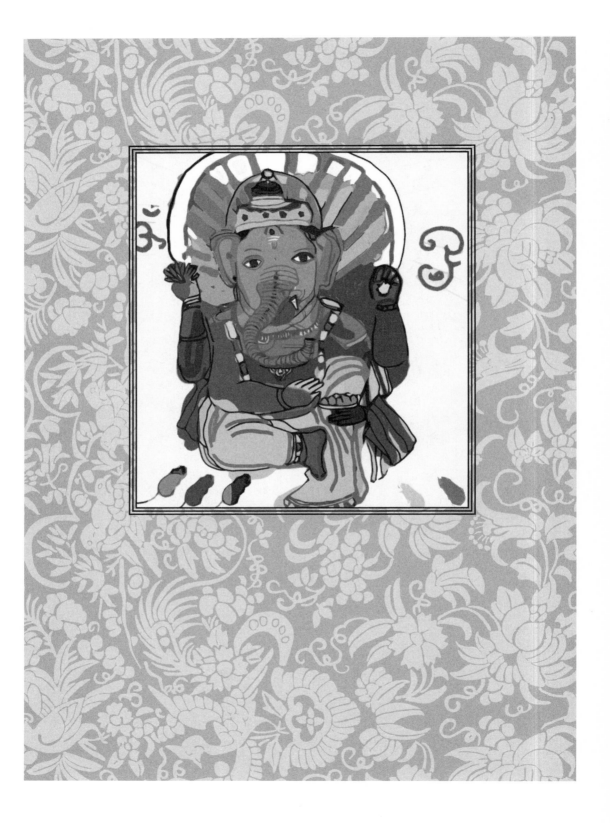

YOGA
for Stuttering

*Unifying the Voice, Breath,
Mind & Body to
Achieve Fluent Speech*

J. M. BALAKRISHNAN

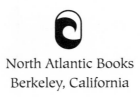

North Atlantic Books
Berkeley, California

Published by   Cover art, photographs, and artwork by Josephine Balakrishnan
North Atlantic Books   Cover and book design by Suzanne Albertson
P.O. Box 12327
Berkeley, California 94712   Printed in the United States of America

Illustration on page 10 © iStockphoto.com/Vasiliy Yakobchuk; illustration on page 11 © iStockphoto.com/Sebastian Kaulitzki; illustration on page 64 © iStockphoto.com/Eduard Härkönen; photograph on page 64 © iStockphoto.com/Xyno; photograph on page 65 © iStockphoto.com/Dmitry Rukhlenko; photograph on page 65 © iStockphoto.com/Manuela Krause

Yoga for Stuttering: Unifying the Voice, Breath, Mind & Body to Achieve Fluent Speech is sponsored by the Society for the Study of Native Arts and Sciences, a nonprofit educational corporation whose goals are to develop an educational and cross-cultural perspective linking various scientific, social, and artistic fields; to nurture a holistic view of arts, sciences, humanities, and healing; and to publish and distribute literature on the relationship of mind, body, and nature.

North Atlantic Books' publications are available through most bookstores. For further information, visit our Web site at www.northatlanticbooks.com or call 800-733-3000.

Library of Congress Cataloging-in-Publication Data

Balakrishnan, J.M. (Josephine M.)
   Yoga for stuttering : unifying the voice, breath, mind & body to achieve fluent speech / J.M. Balakrishnan.
        p. cm.
   Includes bibliographical references and index.
   ISBN 978-1-55643-768-7
1. Hatha yoga—Therapeutic use. 2. Stuttering—Alternative treatment. I. Title.
   RM727.Y64B35 2009
   613.7'046—dc22   2008049009

1 2 3 4 5 6 7 8 9 SHERIDAN 14 13 12 11 10 09

To Sri Mata Amritanandamayi

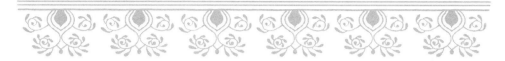

Contents

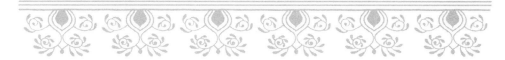

Preface

"Man is made by his belief. As he believes, so he is."
—BHAGAVAD GITA

One of my consistent nightmares as a child was picking up a phone only to find that I couldn't speak. In these dreams I would put my hand to my face and find that there were bandages around my mouth. Perhaps this is why I spent my life studying communication. After studying acting and public speaking in high school, I became a champion debater and public speaker in college. I won national awards and debated for the University of California, Berkeley. I obtained my master's in speech communication from California State University, San Francisco, and did doctoral work in speech communication at Pennsylvania State University. I obtained a law degree with the ambition of becoming a trial lawyer; however, I found myself more fascinated by speech than by law.

Leo Tolstoy opens the tragic novel *Anna Karenina,* "Happy families are all alike; every unhappy family is unhappy in its own way." Similarly, I found that the strengths of good speakers were comparable, yet each unsuccessful speaker experienced unique problems. The differences were interesting to me; I enjoyed unraveling speaking problems. I went on to obtain my master's in communicative disorders from California State University, Northridge, and became a licensed speech pathologist.

For more than twenty-five years I have worked with a wide range of students in over one hundred schools. I helped them with a variety of speech communication problems, from difficulty producing one phoneme (a unit of sound) to an inability to communicate on any level. However, disfluency—as stuttering is called—mystified me. I was not happy with the therapy methods provided for my students who stuttered. I wanted them to succeed, but—despite exhaustive research—I found few methods that met my students' needs.

Most of the boys I saw were very verbal in elementary school despite their stutter, but became self-conscious in middle school, and generally stopped talking by the time they were in high school. The girls stopped talking sooner, as early as elementary school, and often were not identified as having a speech problem, and subsequently were not referred for speech therapy. I saw the devastating effects on students who had no remediation; I remember in particular two girls who were referred to me as selectively mute. In fact, they simply stuttered and would attempt to speak only at home. I spent years searching for a program to help these students.

Some studies suggest that stuttering is primarily an emotional issue; the speaker becomes stressed at the possibility of stuttering, and subsequently continues to stutter. Many researchers have noticed that bad feedback from others actually inspires more stuttering. This was my understanding when I met Larry and Harry (not their real names, although their names did rhyme), two charming young twins who filled the room with their excitement and energy as soon as they entered. Larry and Harry stuttered but were not subdued like my other students. Their energy was so high they could have accomplished any task put in front of them. I think they understood I was ill-equipped to help them and decided to have fun with me. Larry would run to the window and pull the shutter up and down rapidly while Harry rattled off a series of questions at me, and then Larry would interrupt and ask me another set. Neither of them ever stopped stuttering.

The boys showed me how stuttering occurs. I could see how they were speaking. Most students were self-conscious, which further impaired their ability to speak clearly. Larry and Harry's exuberance indicated their stuttering was not emotional. It was due to their speech mechanism. Because there were two of them I could better observe the context in which they stuttered. There didn't seem to be specific sounds that they struggled with, or ideas that were hard for them to express. They weren't stuttering because they were worried they might. This was new information that had not been considered in most research. I began to look more closely at the speech mechanism.

I learned more from my friend George, a graphic designer, who had had a severe stutter. He would be fluent for long periods but then would descend into long stretches of stuttering. Each word took a long time to produce, and his sentences became so fragmented it was difficult to follow what he was trying to say. He tried every approach, including hypnosis and drug therapy, and spent hundreds of thousands of dollars going to specialists. He even married a speech therapist! The only thing that helped him was a mantra given to him by his teacher. Fifteen years ago, I had little knowledge of what a mantra was.

George's success fascinated me. What was a mantra? Was it a religious belief? Why would a mantra work better than any other method? Did mantras have magical power? I did some research and found that, in the East Indian tradition, a mantra is a sound that evokes specific vibrations. These sounds, primarily one syllable, represent large concepts connected to philosophical beliefs but not necessarily religious in nature. The core of a mantra is the vibrations that are produced. I learned that *aum,* also spelled *ohm* and *om,* was a mantra, possibly akin to "amen."

In a particularly stressful moment, I asked a five-year-old student to say "aum" to see if it helped his stutter. He told me that it "made his heart feel good." He didn't stutter during that session. I was shocked since I knew he didn't have a preconceived notion of the effect of the mantra. However, since I worked in public schools, I wondered about the practicality of requiring students to chant "aum." In the United States, separation of church and state prohibits public schools from providing religious instruction, directing religious activity, or restricting personal religious expression, but schools may teach about religion. Although several Eastern religions share the symbology of aum, it is not a concept specific to religion; however, I felt it might be misconstrued in a school setting. I envisioned a court case where I lost.

I went home and stewed over my dilemma. There was a knock at my door. My neighbor, Martha, came to my rescue by pointing out that worldwide, all vowels are considered mantras. I found she was right. There is a long tradition of vowels being used in sacred and therapeutic singing.[1] I could work with vowels. I found a large body of research indicating that historically it has not been unusual for medical doctors to incorporate sound, singing, and chanting as part of a cure.[2]

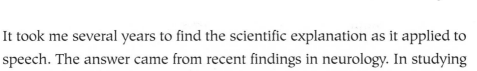

It took me several years to find the scientific explanation as it applied to speech. The answer came from recent findings in neurology. In studying the brain, scientists have found that speech is controlled by two areas in the left hemisphere. Singing, meanwhile, is controlled by the right hemisphere.

It is an interesting phenomenon: most people who stutter do not stutter when singing. New medical studies have found that in those who stutter, the neurological pathways in the left hemisphere of the brain are stronger than in the right hemisphere.[3] Neurologists have found that when stroke patients are unable to access their speech, they can be taught to speak again by the use of prolonged utterances.[4] Slow singing—melodic intonation—has been successful in building neurological pathways. Scientists conclude that developing the left hemisphere of the brain also develops the right hemisphere. It follows that stuttering can be improved by a similar method. A mantra is a prolonged utterance produced by the right hemisphere of the brain. As the right brain develops neurological pathways, the left brain compensates. This closes the loop, and the speaking mechanism is improved. Finally I had a scientific basis to show why chanting and mantras help stuttering.

Yoga for Stuttering is a combination of Yoga methods that rely on these findings. I have used these methods, and they have been successful with a variety of students. The fastest progress was a high school student who worked hard and cleared his stutter in two weeks. As with any method, I recommend incorporating these exercises into another daily routine, such as brushing your teeth, showering, or driving. Consistency leads to change.

If this method is practiced diligently you will see results. Fortunately, most people who stutter are motivated.

J. M. BALAKRISHNAN, MA, MS, JD
Albany, California

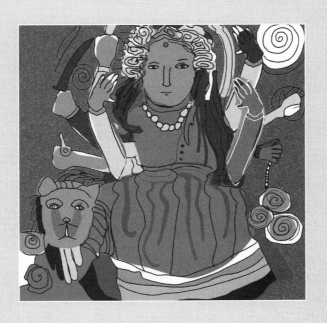

PART 1
Yoga for Stuttering

"The meaning of our self is not to be found in its separateness from God and others, but in the ceaseless realization of yoga, of union."

—RABINDRANATH TAGORE

Yoga for Stuttering combines the results of recent studies in neurology with three branches of Yoga: Hatha (union through movement), Nada (union through sound), and Raja (union through thought). Neurological research shows that stimulating the left hemisphere of the brain affects the right hemisphere in compensation. The reverse is also true: singing and chanting to activate the right hemisphere affects the speech processes of the left hemisphere. Yoga for Stuttering joins this scientific model with an ancient discipline to increase fluent speech.

You do not have to have any knowledge of Yoga to practice this method. The *Yoga for Stuttering* workbook uses photos and illustrations to make it easy to work independently on fluency. Yoga for Stuttering can also be used with a speech pathologist trained in this method. Each pose in this book is presented in three parts, with opening stories intended as guidance for Raja meditation, followed by a Hatha Yoga posture, and finally an exercise that lets you practice making the sounds of Nada Yoga.

Although Hatha, Nada, and Raja Yoga have long been used in Asia for remediation, in the West we are just beginning to explore possible applications. The Yoga for Stuttering method was created to meet the needs of those who stutter who have not been able to obtain relief through traditional methods, as well as those who want to try a different approach.

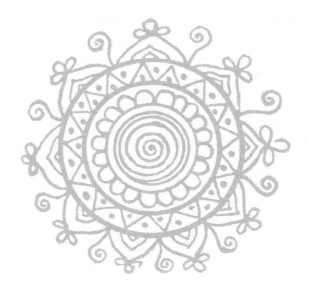

1

Who Stutters and Why

Sixty million adults in the world stutter. Only five percent of them, or three million people, are actually identified by therapists as having a stutter. Of those who seek therapy, eighty percent are able to increase fluency, but twenty percent continue to search for help.[6] These numbers are alarming. Three million people are severely impaired by their inability to produce clear, fluent speech. Although myriad theories exist to explain why some people are fluent and some aren't, there is no agreed upon conclusion. No one is fluent all of the time. Some people start stuttering later in life. We do know that stuttering runs in families, and that the majority of those afflicted are male. Some researchers argue stuttering is genetic, some claim it's a result of environmental factors, and others consider it a physical limitation. Most researchers agree that stuttering comes and goes, but, if unaddressed, after a certain age emotional and psychological issues can seriously affect the person who stutters.

Case Study: Brenda— Expanding Confidence

In the 1990s I was a speech therapist in one of the lowest performing high schools in California. One of my students, Brenda, didn't speak. I had to hunt through the different records throughout her schooling to determine why she was assigned to a speech therapist. My supervisor reviewed Brenda's history and told me to dismiss her because she appeared to be "selectively mute." "Selective mutism" is an anxiety disorder that inhibits speech. Because it is not an inability to speak due to a physical impediment, it is therefore not within the domain of a speech therapist, but would typically be addressed by a psychologist.[25] Brenda's teachers did not feel she needed counseling but insisted she needed speech therapy. I researched her case and found that early on she had been identified as a person who stutters. I met with Brenda to determine if speech therapy would help her.

I had to determine why Brenda wasn't speaking. Her records showed that she had stopped talking at school around age ten. Brenda's mother came to see me. She told me this was a family pattern. As a child, she herself had also not spoken in public. Brenda's mother was difficult to understand because she spoke in a soft, often inaudible voice.

After a few sessions with Brenda, it was difficult to understand what was going on. She did not seem depressed, yet she never spoke. I talked for most of the session and noted her nonverbal responses: nodding her head, smiling, etc. I was confused by her ability to engage without speaking. I was ready to refer Brenda to a psychologist when she started speaking. Her voice was very soft. She revealed she was worried that she would stutter so she was careful about whom she spoke to. She said she didn't stutter with everyone. Brenda had narrowed her communicative world to her family and close friends with whom she felt relaxed. She did stutter with them but not as often as she feared she might with strangers. One of her biggest phobias was answering the phone.

My challenge as a speech therapist was to help Brenda expand her world. As an assignment, I had her call offices to get information about colleges that she might attend. She reported back that she had been very nervous and had continued to stutter, but she had accomplished the task. I was happy that she had built up trust with me, but the fact remained that she needed to be able to communicate comfortably in order to complete her education and maintain a vocation. Brenda needed a new solution in a world in which communication is critical. I pointed out that if she were asked out on a date and couldn't reply, she would be losing out. She laughed, and agreed to practice.

Because Brenda spoke so softly, when we began Yoga for Stuttering one of the goals was to use vocal exercises to increase her volume. With a bit more focus on her voice, she came to realize the more she used it the better it sounded. At first she was squeaky, like a trumpet that hasn't been played for a while. Gradually she gained power in her voice. This helped her fluency. Brenda became more pleased with the sound of her voice and less critical. A key factor in fluency is knowing the range of your voice. Yoga for Stuttering exercises are similar to dance routines. A dancer knows what his body can do, and when he is able to extend his movement, rather than being held back by fear, he can accomplish an elaborate step. Similarly, once Brenda knew she could produce smooth, prolonged sounds, and that she had the breath capacity to keep going if she did stutter, she was able to try. Brenda had to work on both vocal quality and disfluency. Because she had trouble fitting in the exercises with her very large homework load, I suggested that she add one vocal exercise (the Lion) to her normal routines: brushing her teeth, taking a shower, or walking to school. This worked for her.

By our last three sessions, she was rarely disfluent, and was within the norm for the general population. Brenda has since gone to college and continues to use these techniques to build up confidence as well as physical skill. She can now communicate with people she doesn't know, which had been a big challenge for her.

Causes

Stuttering can originate from problems with the neurological system. The brain sends a message through the nervous system, which is not in line with the muscles that control speech. In severe forms this is labeled apraxia of speech. The brain sends a delayed message to the body, and this can cause subsequent jerkiness in physical movements, including speech.

Stuttering can be a product of emotional stress. When the body is in distress, adrenaline is released to speed up the body's response to meet the impending danger—the fight-or-flight response. The brain shoots off quick signals, and, for some, this decreases the efficiency of the speech mechanism. The anxiety of trying to stop a stutter creates another layer of distress, so that being extremely aware of one's stuttering can actually induce more stuttering.

Case Study: David— Creating Channels in the Audio Realm

Often secondary behaviors accompany stuttering. Some are physical manifestations—twitching, scratching, blinking, or head jerking—and some are intentional and creative methods of communicating nonverbally. David was a sixteen-year-old high school student at a high-achieving public school. He was labeled selectively mute; however, his mother requested speech therapy for his stuttering. David was fascinating because he had worked out hundreds of adaptations to communicate. He said he was fine. David was a remarkable student; he wrote, made eye contact, and expressed himself in every way except vocally. He didn't speak to me for several months; however, he did communicate. He used pantomime, including a wide range of facial expressions, to avoid speaking. He carried several journals with him in which to correspond with his friends and teachers.

I wasn't sure how I could help David if he was happy only expressing himself nonverbally. I introduced him to the Yoga for Stuttering method. He practiced the exercises and started talking. He stuttered, but because he felt comfortable opening up to me and being disfluent in front of me, I was able to help him understand that he could speak even if he stuttered. As he practiced Yoga for Stuttering he felt more competent to speak and his disfluency diminished.

David and Brenda (my student described on page 6) had many similarities; they were the same age, both were considered selectively mute, and both were open to trying different methods to overcome their stuttering—including practicing the Yoga for Stuttering methods. Somehow, building up different channels of communication gave them room to explore other methods. Brenda was very sensitive to gestures, movements, and looks. David could have been a pantomime. They showed me that it is possible to function using alternative forms of communication. Their resilience was remarkable; they each found ways of going around—rather than up against—their hurdle.

Although the strength exhibited by creating alternative methods of communication is to be commended, there are many instances in which speaking is expected. Particularly in situations when an explanation is required, a compromise needs to be made, or you need to fight a parking ticket, verbal communication facilitates a quick resolution. Because he did not speak, David's teachers assumed his behavior was due to emotional problems. David did not realize that his extreme behavior was impeding his development, and was impacting not only how others perceived him, but also what he was willing to accept because he could not ensure he was well understood. David is now in college, studying creative writing. He has a girlfriend and is happy. His voice is still soft, but he made great progress by speaking and increasing his ability to use speech.

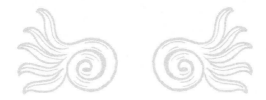

Standard Approaches to Disfluency

Historically some very gruesome methods have been attempted to stop stuttering, including burning the tongue, scarring the throat, and cutting off part of the tongue.[7] Today, there are computer programs, chips for the ear, prescription drugs, and training programs that use a variety of techniques. These programs have generated some successes, but not for everyone, and the cost can be prohibitive. These various methods have contributed to the twelve million people in the United States who have overcome stuttering. However, there are still three million people who need another approach.

New Studies of the Brain

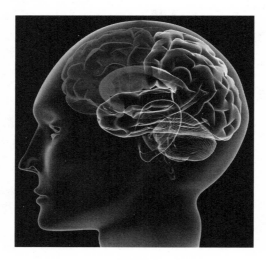

The brain

In 1973, neurological researchers R. W. Sparks, N. A. Helm, and M. L. Albert, while working with adults in the Aphasia Research Unit at the Boston Veterans Administration Hospital, developed a program of singsong, chant-like phrases, which they titled Melodic Intonation Therapy.[8] They found that in stroke patients who had lost their ability to speak, exercising the right hemisphere of the brain compensated for the damage in the left hemisphere.[9]

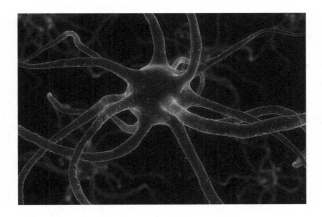

Neuron in the brain

Singing uses the right hemisphere of the brain. Speaking uses the left hemisphere. Most people who stutter do not stutter when singing. Some researchers conjecture the impairment exists primarily in the left hemisphere. Through the use of a series of chants—the prolonged utterances that make up the core of Nada Yoga—the Yoga for Stuttering method works by cross training the brain. If the speaker's ability to produce a prolonged sound is increased, a set of parallel skills is developed which enables the speaker to speak fluently.

Singing has already been used to remedy speech. Vocal exercises are standard therapy for many speech impediments.[10] We can extend this to stuttering and see that using a set of prolonged utterances will improve a speaker's fluency.[11]

Case Study: Mary—Centering

Mary was a tall young woman who seemed shy, but replied fluently when questioned. She had long hair and her ears were pierced with vivid yellow sapphire earrings. Her dress was a tiny set of pleats. She appeared to be very tidy. Everything was in place. Mary was also very creative, and liked drawing and painting. After I explained the principle behind Yoga for Stuttering, I could feel her resistance. She said she didn't think it would work. I told her about the area of the brain that contains the neurological pathways that control the speech mechanism, and about the functions of the left and right hemispheres. I wanted to show her that I had developed this method based on neurological studies, and not simply because I liked Yoga. She nodded thoughtfully. After many sessions, Mary explained that one of her problems was that everyone said she should relax, but that she felt she was a relaxed person. She didn't consider her disfluency to be a product of nervousness.

As a speech therapist, I focus on every aspect of communication. Words are only one component of speech. In Mary's case, she saw Yoga only as a method of relaxation—and she found relaxation techniques stressful since she felt they were a waste of time. Yoga's focus on deep breathing contributes to its reputation as a relaxation method. Mary felt that she didn't need to relax. And, speaking to her, I didn't feel tension except at her resistance to the concept. Her resistance was linked to the fact that, despite the numerous programs she had been through since she was very young, she was still a severe stutterer.

Resistance to relaxation is something I can identify with. The underlying concept is that there isn't enough time. In fact, stuttering can be seen as a problem with the concept of time. When Mary wanted to speak, she was stopped, she was told to slow down, and she was told to relax. In her mind, she was being asked to waste the very thing that she found to be in short supply: time. She wanted to be efficient; she wanted to speak easily and quickly.

Albert Einstein introduced time as a relative concept. He explained, "When a man sits with a pretty girl for an hour, it seems like a minute. But let him sit on a hot stove for a minute and it's longer than any hour. That's relativity." The Hopi Indians do not have a past, present, or future in their language. Time is a form we place on top of what we are doing to evaluate and compromise. Having an agreed-upon record of time establishes order and generally works to our advantage. Clocks all show the same numbers, but we may experience time differently; sometimes it is "running fast," other times it is "running slow." People who stutter often experience their heart racing and their blood pumping in their effort to communicate. For them, precious time is running out; their listeners are giving them constant signals that they want to end the communication.

Mary resisted giving control of time to someone else. She described her disfluency as something that had a life of its own, that wasn't connected to her. The thought of relaxing and potentially releasing this animal that might consume her was very stressful.

Let's take a closer look at Mary and her beliefs. She believed she didn't have enough time and that relaxing would take more time. Since time is relative, being relaxed or tense is not a major factor in evaluating how long it takes to complete a task. What Mary needed to examine was whether her concept of time was based in reality. If you want to speak faster, will it help to tell yourself you're not speaking fast enough? Mary and I decided to explore this further. I asked her to pick a task she was concerned about, one for which she felt she needed more time. Mary decided to examine whether she could do her homework faster if she relaxed and didn't look at the clock, or if she repeatedly told herself to hurry up and reminded herself that she didn't have enough time. Mary reported back that she worked faster without the reminder, and made fewer mistakes.

We then extended that to her speech. I suggested she tell herself during the next disfluent moment to go faster and see if she stuttered less. Also, because—for Mary—saying "relax" was invoking "go faster," we created a new statement: "I can push the edge of time." She adjusted her relationship to time by imagining being in a bubble. She could then push the edges—in this bubble she could relax because she had all the time she needed. This concept enabled Mary to try the Yoga for Stuttering method.

Studies from the East

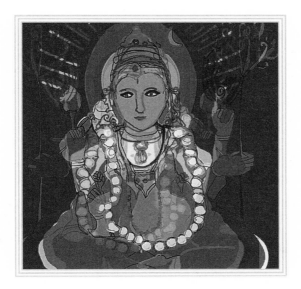

East Indian research has long used deep breathing and physical exercises to reduce stuttering. Although Yoga is known in the West primarily as a set of physical postures (Hatha Yoga or asanas), this is only one form of Yoga. Yoga is a Sanskrit word meaning "union." Nada Yoga, union through sound, is used to improve speech through prolonged utterances, mantras, and chants designed to "tune the inner body." Raja refers to the meditative techniques used to focus the mind. Raja, Hatha, and Nada Yoga overlap. The union of these three branches of Yoga is the foundation of Yoga for Stuttering: strengthening and coordinating both the brain and the muscles of the body.[12]

2

Yoga Philosophy

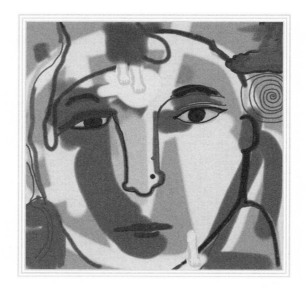

Indian philosophy holds that through disciplined study a person may obtain liberation from all suffering. The world is considered to be full of distractions. Yoga is the name of the training to overcome those distractions. There are many schools of Yoga incorporating meditation, movement, and voice into virtually every aspect of living. Raja Yoga is an ancient school of meditation. Hatha Yoga, the study of body positions to enhance physical agility, is the branch of Yoga most of us are familiar with in the West. Nada Yoga, the study of sound, is not as well known in this country. This form of Yoga uses drills and practices to discipline the mind through the training of the voice and ear.[13] Nada Yoga exercises involve producing a clear, accurate tone with prolonged utterances usually involving vowels and semivowels such as diphthongs.

Raja Yoga

The foundation of Raja Yoga is meditation: increasing focus through mental concentration. Raja Yogis hold that it is the royal Yoga above all other forms of Yoga—without it, it is difficult not only to achieve the proper postures required for asanas, but also to produce and hear clear sound. Without conquering the mind, little physical progress can be made.[14]

Neurologists are learning more about the brain's ability to grow and change as new technologies reveal an abundance of connections in the brain. Previously, the brain was considered to be fully developed by adulthood, and to decay with age. Current studies, however, show the brain's flexibility and its potential to be retrained. Recently there have been studies documenting the positive effects of various meditative techniques.[15]

Raja Yoga is a Yoga of the mind, a training of the mind through mental focus. There are many ways to train the mind, by studying books and through the act of meditation; often, deep insights arise from a combination of both. To perform Raja Yoga meditation as an ongoing spiritual practice, it is important to have a teacher. To find a teacher, consult the resources listed on page 101. However, in order to benefit from the Raja Yoga exercises in this book to improve your vocal fluency, you only need to have an attitude of openness to the effect of the exercises.

To practice the meditation, sit on a chair or cross-legged on the floor with your back straight, the palms of your hands resting lightly on your lap or your knees. Breathe long deep breaths until your breath is flowing easily. Focus inwardly on your breath and follow the directions outlined under each of the Yoga exercises in part 3 of this book.

Hatha Yoga in Rehabilitation

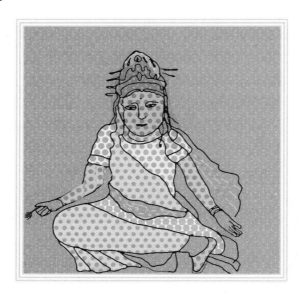

Hatha Yoga is effective as a method for improving muscle tone and has been used to treat numerous ailments, from heart disease to neurosis. In a one-year controlled study examining the effect of Yoga as a therapeutic tool for people with cognitive disabilities, researchers found significant improvement in social adaptation and attention span, as well as improvements in physical skills and coordination. Extensive studies show that Yoga can reduce anxiety and hostility, improve depression, and, specifically, improve a speaker's fluency.[16]

A vital aspect of Hatha Yoga is awareness of breath. While breathing is automatic, it is also an action we can practice consciously.[17] Breath control has long been considered an important part of healing. There are many books that describe the function of the breath and its effect on anxiety and depression.[18]

Breathing is so simple and obvious we often take it for granted, ignoring its power to affect body, mind, and spirit. With each inhale we bring oxygen into the body, and with each exhale we purge the body of carbon dioxide, a toxic waste. Breathing affects our state of mind. It can make us excited or calm, tense or relaxed. It can make our thinking confused or clear. In the yogic tradition, air is the primary source of *prana,* or "life force"—a psycho-physio-spiritual force that permeates the universe.

Pranayama is loosely translated as "life energy through breathing." Yogis have developed a series of breathing techniques to control life energy as it moves through the body. Pranayama is used in Yoga as a separate practice to help clear and cleanse the body and mind. It is also used in preparation for meditation, and in asana (the practice of postures) to help maximize the benefits of the practice and focus the mind.[19]

Nada Yoga

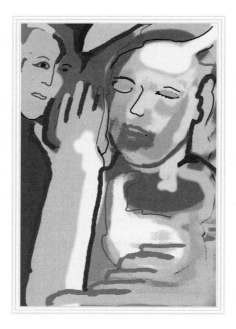

In Sanskrit *nada* means "sound." Indian music concentrates on obtaining clarity in sound. The focus of the musician or singer is to perfect each note. To Western ears these notes seem slow and prolonged. To the Indian ear, Western music sounds noisy, full of disharmony and interruption.[20]

One essential element of Nada Yoga is the vowel. Vowels cause the speaker to produce a clear stream of air without obstruction because they are open-ended. The human body resonates the open sound.[21]

Strengthening the ability to produce prolonged sounds increases vocal power. The ability to intentionally produce short staccato sounds increases the power to rewire the speaking mechanism, resulting in fewer involuntary staccato utterances. Strengthening one side of the brain strengthens the other. Various exercise and training systems are based on this concept. Cross-lateral movements increase strength in opposing sides. This can also be seen in the body's constant efforts to maintain balance. At the brain level, attention-deficit disorder (ADD) is a good example. With ADD, ability to hyper-focus often goes hand in hand with the general disability to sift, prioritize, and pay attention. Hyper-focusing for long periods of time further weakens the mind's ability to focus generally.

Melodic Intonation Therapy (MIT) is very similar to Nada Yoga training exercises. Both work toward producing prolonged utterances in a tone sequence. MIT has been used successfully since the 1970s. Although MIT is used worldwide for aphasia and has been recently applied to apraxia, it is also being used as speech therapy for disfluency. In a related study, Nicki Cohen has conducted studies of singing and its effect on rehabilitating the speech production of neurologically impaired persons.[22] She found that singing three times a week for three weeks caused a significant improvement in the participants of her study. Sixty-seven percent of those in the study improved their speaking range, tone, and quality, as well as their rate of speech.

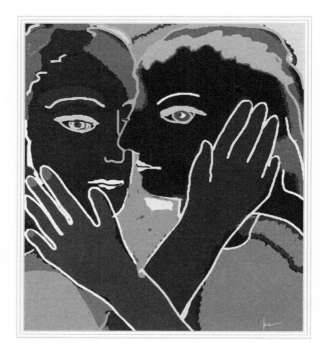

Hatha Yoga has been used in physical therapy, and has rehabilitated many of the muscles used in speech production. Nada Yoga, however, has not been studied as remediation but has mainly been used as a tool for developing professional vocal qualities. Although lay practitioners use chanting to improve breathing and vocal quality, there is a scarcity of research in this area.[23] However, given that Hatha and Nada Yoga can be used to improve overall intelligibility, it is likely that future scientific studies will show a strong correlation between Yoga and fluency.[24]

Case study: Harry—
Swimming with the Flow

Harry, a young man in his twenties, felt angry that he was discriminated against because of his disfluency. He was constantly upset that the world was not more sensitive to his needs. Stuttering became part of his identity. Harry had a series of valid complaints. He felt he should be allowed more time to complete the oral exams required to advance in his workplace, and more time to respond to questions in general; he believed that listeners should be required by law to listen to him without interrupting. He felt discriminated against at work because his boss would constantly cut him off and not let him start speaking because he was worried that Harry's response would take too long. He protested that just as there is designated parking for handicapped people, the telephone company should give him a break on long-distance calls. And women wouldn't give him the time of day. When he came to see me, I could only listen and try to be sensitive to his position, but his anger was not helping. I explained to him that since neither he nor I can easily change the outside world to suit his needs, perhaps an alternative method, Yoga for Stuttering, might help him adjust. Harry agreed to try speech therapy.

For someone who stutters, there may be a false sense that everyone else in the rest of the world is fluent. I explained to Harry it wasn't helpful to see things from an either-or perspective; I advised him to stop identifying himself as a stutterer, and everyone else as fluent. In fact, most people stutter. It's common for people to speak with hesitations, pauses, and shakiness. Just as life is never black-and-white, neither is the ability to communicate. Perceiving the potential for understanding is a very important part of being human, and is the basis for communication. Without communication we feel vulnerable, and stuttering can be the result. I wanted Harry to be aware that his anger represented his fear of being unable to communicate. And, rather than direct-ing his energy as anger at the world, he could direct it toward improving under-standing.

I suggested to Harry that rather than insisting the world adapt, he exam-ine how he had adapted thus far, and how that was evidence of his ability to communicate. Harry needed to acknowledge his accomplishments: he was a member of a forum for disfluency, he was a great writer, he loved to sing, and he was generally fluent among certain people. There are few people who always stutter, and the amount of time stuttering changes from day to day, situation to situation, minute to minute.

Harry was reluctant to see himself as within the norm. Instead he stated, "Why have I been discriminated against at work?" "Why did the girl I like drop me?" All kinds of people lose jobs, and girlfriends. He had to come to terms with the fact that stuttering does not preclude success; after all, Tiger Woods, a person who stuttered, has had no problem with his career. "Stutter" is a rel-ative term. What *is* constant and consistent is the fear of stuttering. But it is just as true that we might not stutter as that we might stutter. Harry didn't understand the fear I was referring to. I explained that I was asking him only to look at his basic underlying idea that he couldn't communicate, and see if that was true. Harry had been trying to control his environment to adapt to his disfluency. He was in constant pain because he couldn't control those around him.

Harry was suddenly quiet. He then started recalling times when he had been fluent: when he spoke to his friend while they fished, when he asked to borrow something from a neighbor, when he sang in the chorus. "It comes and goes," he noted. Once he recognized that he was fluent more often than he thought, he understood that Yoga for Stuttering was a tool he could use to increase his fluency.

I explained to Harry that the Lion exercises focus on the power of the world. *Srimat simhasanasvari,* the third mantra in the sacred twelfth-century Indian text *Sri Lalita Sahasranama,* refers to the two lions who protect the power of the world. These are the lions of the Simhasana (Lion pose). We each have a source of power that we draw from. I asked Harry to look at that power. He was able to see that turning fear into anger was not effective. And he was able to address his own fear of not being able to communicate, to persevere in his attempts to be more fluent, and to accept that he will never be able to control the way people react to him.

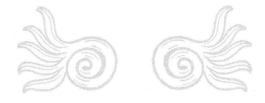

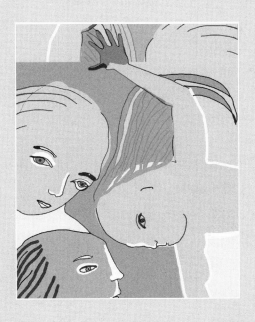

PART 2
The Method

*"Yoga teaches us to cure what need not be endured
and endure what cannot be cured."*

—B. K. S. IYENGAR

Yoga for Stuttering combines exercises from the three types of Yoga discussed in this book. If these exercises are practiced you will improve vocal fluency (decrease stuttering) and:

Increase the power of your breath

Strengthen the muscles used in speaking

Produce rapid, accurate, coordinated articulation

Control airflow and increase voice quality

Increase attention and focus

Diminish interfering thoughts

Each of the following lessons can be done independently or in combination. Each segment of the program incorporates the unified principles of Yoga: Hatha (physical postures), Nada (vocal exercises), and Raja (meditative practices).

If you haven't done any Yoga previously, practice one asana (position) until you feel comfortable, and than add the next. Start by practicing for ten minutes a day, then increase the amount of time each day. If you have difficulty with any of these positions, or are ready for more advanced positions, a licensed Yoga instructor should be able to help you.

The American Yoga Association Web site can help you find a teacher in your area. Yoga for Stuttering is a speech therapy program, and if you are having difficulty with speech production you may need the help of a speech pathologist. You can find referrals on the American Speech-Language-Hearing Association Web site (see the resources listed on page 101 toward the end of this book).

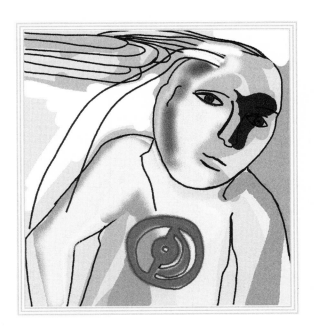

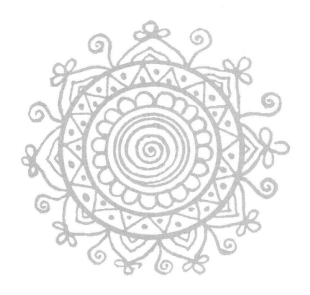

3

Exercises

Exercise 1. Initial Assessment

GOAL: Record an inventory of the rate of your speech.

Record how long you can produce a vowel (see chart). Record how long you can hold a smooth continuous sound with only one breath (do not take small sips of air to continue as you might while singing). This is the "before" measurement.

Please note that unless you have been singing or practicing, your voice will probably not be smooth at this beginning point. This would be a challenge even if you did not have a stutter. However, with practice, your voice will become smooth and your breath control will improve.

Initial Assessment			Date:	
Speaking		Singing (choose a note and hold it)		
Sound (pronunciation guide is given in parentheses)	**Duration (seconds)**	**Sound** (pronunciation guide is given in parentheses)	**Duration (seconds)**	
a (ah)		a (ah)		
A (*a*ngel)		A (*a*ngel)		
E (eee)		E (eee)		
I (eye)		I (eye)		
O (ok)		O (ok)		
oo (moon)		oo (moon)		

Exercise 2. Progress

GOAL: Increase the length of time and tone of your production of open vowels.

You may fill in this worksheet on a daily or a weekly basis. The more often you practice, the faster you will improve, and it is helpful to keep a regular routine. As you practice, remain aware of the relative ease with which you produce the notes as well as the length and timbre of your chanting. On some days it will be harder to produce a prolonged utterance; on others, it will be easier. Try not to judge your performance but simply observe how your voice changes from day to day.

Progress		Date:	
Speaking		**Singing**	
Sound	**Duration (seconds)**	**Sound**	**Duration (seconds)**
a (ah)		a (ah)	
A (*a*ngel)		A (*a*ngel)	
E (eee)		E (eee)	
I (eye)		I (eye)	
O (ok)		O (ok)	
oo (moon)		oo (moon)	

Excercise 3. Fine Tuning

GOAL: Feel the vibration of vowels within five parts of the body.

There are successful musicians who cannot hear with their ears; instead they feel the sound with other parts of their body. These exercises will help you feel the vibrations of vowels. The five parts of the body used in Yoga for Stuttering to feel sound vibration are the crown, forehead, throat, chest, and gut.

We have learned a lot from those who are deaf. Evelyn Glennie is perhaps the best-known deaf musician. She is an award-winning percussionist who performs all over the world. Her speaking voice is lyrical and tonal. She states that she hears vibrations with her body.

This lesson is designed to increase our sensitivity to our own voice in the rest of our body. For the purposes of this program, do not evaluate your stutter, but the quality of the vowel tone. The important part is to feel the differences in the vibration of each sound. Place your hand over each of the five parts of the body as you produce each vowel.

The crown: In a newborn baby this area is not yet fused. It is soft. Gradually the skull becomes fused, except for an area on top of your skull where you can feel vibrations more profoundly. You can feel vibrations in this area by placing your hand on the top of your head or a bit above it.

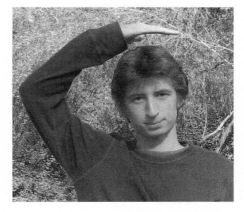

The forehead: The forehead has an area above the bridge of the nose where it is easy to feel sound vibrations.

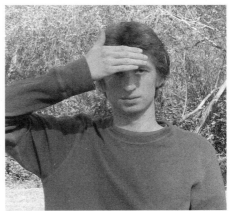

The front of your throat: Some deaf people learn speech by putting their hands on the speaker's throat. Needless to say, this isn't something that can be done with strangers. However, the vibrations of specific phonemes (units of sound) are easier to distinguish in this area.

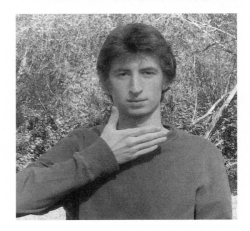

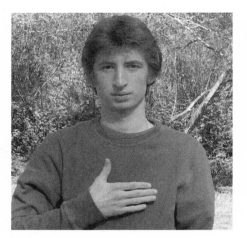

The chest bone: This area is my favorite. For a time I would place my hands over this spot and find it immediately soothing. It is easy to feel the vibration of sound here.

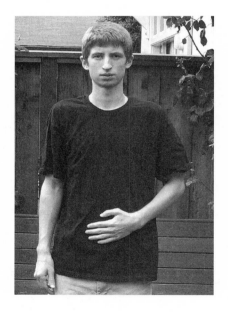

The gut: A bit below the navel, this area has a very low, deep resonance. Martial artists often produce vocalizations from this area.

Record your reactions in each part of the body.

Physical Reactions				Date:	
Sound (pronunciation guide is given in parentheses)	Head	Throat	Chest	Gut	Legs
a (ah)					
A (*a*ngel)					
E (eee)					
I (eye)					
O (ok)					
oo (moon)					

Here is an example of what you might note down:

Sound	Head	Throat	Chest	Gut	Legs
a (ah)	strong	faint	loud	hard to do	can't feel it

Exercise 4. Journaling

GOAL: Choose vowels and use overtones.

This is a good exercise for those who like visual imagery. You can choose to work with all the vowels, but most students have found that they are attached to one or two vowels. The goal is to practice expanding the length of your vocalizations and to concentrate on the sound in each of the five areas of your body. Visualize moving the sound from one part of the body to another.

Sound Journal		Date:
Sound (pronunciation guide is given in parentheses)	**Perceptions**	
a (ah)		
A (*a*ngel)		
E (eee)		
I (eye)		
O (ok)		
oo (moon)		

Here is an example of how you might record your perceptions:

a (ah)	reminds me of air
A (*a*ngel)	my favorite sound

Exercise 5. Singing

GOAL: Sing very slowly.

Create a list of songs that you enjoy singing extremely slowly. One song I love to practice with my students is "Row, Row, Row Your Boat." The concept of the Yoga for Stuttering method is embedded in the lyrics. The song reminds us to be present, in the moment, as if floating down a stream in a boat. The future is unknown, and "life is but a dream."

Row, row, row your boat,
Gently down the stream.
Merrily, merrily, merrily, merrily,
Life is but a dream.

Choose any of your favorite songs, and sing it very, very slowly.

Singing	Date:
Title of Song	

Case Study: Greg—Fluency Flash!

Greg was a fourteen-year-old boy whose family had immigrated to the U.S. from Egypt. His parents did not speak English. Greg had been identified as having a stutter, and for the previous three years he had seen a speech therapist one to two times a week. Yet he still stuttered. He didn't understand at least thirty percent of what was being said; however, he had a friendly personality and was well liked by his friends and the school staff. He was frustrated, but was anxious to succeed. When I first explained the Yoga for Stuttering techniques, he took notes, and when he came back the following week he said he had been practicing his chosen sound. I was impressed since many students find it difficult to stay organized. Particularly in high school, speech therapy can be intrusive on their classes. Greg was motivated by his desire to not be identified as disabled. He worked very hard, and, to both of our amazement, in one month Greg no longer stuttered. I checked on Greg each month and he was completely fluent. I asked, "What was your success due to?" He replied, "I just did what you said."

Greg had listened and tried the Yoga for Stuttering method. Perhaps if he had had more experience he might have resisted as many of us do. However, he picked a vowel and committed to practicing it, which extended his ability to produce prolonged sounds. I was surprised not only at how quickly he improved, but became a fluent, confident speaker.

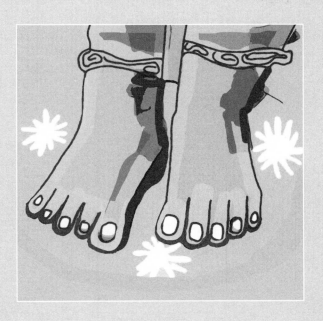

PART 3
The Yoga Exercises

"The power of God is with you at all times; through the activities of mind, senses, breathing, and emotions; and is constantly doing all the work using you as a mere instrument."

—BHAGAVAD GITA

4

The Lion

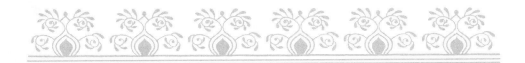

Raja Yoga: Lion

> Once, Lady Peldarbum said to Jetsun Milarepa, "When I meditated on the ocean, my mind was very comfortable. When I meditated on the waves, my mind was troubled. Teach me to meditate on the waves!"
>
> The great Yogi responded, "The waves are the movement of the ocean. Leave them to subside by themselves in its vastness. When you run after your thoughts you are like a dog chasing a stick; every time a stick is thrown, you run after it. But if, instead, you look at where your thoughts are coming from, you will see that each thought arises and dissolves within the space of that awareness, without engendering other thoughts.
>
> "Be like a lion, who, rather than chasing after the stick, turns to face the thrower. You only throw a stick at a lion once."
>
> —*Milarepa, quoted by the late Dilgo Khyentse*[26]

The Lion pose, *Simhasana,* has been used in India for thousands of years as a remedy for stuttering. The posture focuses on deep breathing and speech production, while increasing the strength of the jaw, tongue, throat, neck, chest, and lungs.

A yoga posture is called an *asana* from the Sanskrit word for "seat." The seat of Yoga for Stuttering is the Lion: Simhasana. The Yoga for Stuttering exercises include Hatha, Nada, and Raja segments; Simhasana is a perfect form including all three methods in one posture.

As Milarepa points out in the story above, you cannot throw a stick to confuse or frighten a lion. The lion, unlike a dog or bear, looks to the thrower. If you throw a stick at a dog he runs toward the stick. Bears are confused by sticks thrown at or near them. When coming upon a bear it is good to throw a stick at it. The lion's gaze is similar to a spotlight; it does not get distracted.

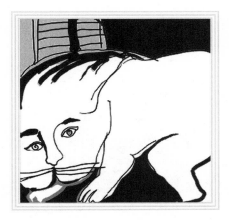

This story is profound. If any of us could look toward ourselves as the lion looks toward us, rather than being distracted by outside circumstances, we would change dramatically. We would not focus on the stick—our thoughts—leading us not to answers but to distraction. For the person who stutters, the "sticks" are thoughts about the stutter.

Some of the thoughts that lead to an inability to speak fluently are those that analyze the meaning of the stutter rather than focusing on communicating to the listener. Here are a few of the possible sticks that the speaker can chase rather than bringing himself back to the task: "Oh no, I'm doing it again, it's not going to stop. I shouldn't have started to speak. I am plagued by this disease. The therapy didn't work. I need help." These thoughts distract the speaker from the task of clear communication, and he finds himself following a succession of sticks that quickly becomes a myriad of splinters.

All speakers stutter. A fluent speaker focuses on producing speech and has the ability to not follow his thoughts about any stutter that appears. Concentrating on the lion's inherent ability to focus is a strong meditation.

"What do you do when the stone lion roars?"
—ZEN BUDDHIST KOAN

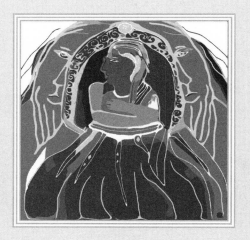

The Shoulder of the Lion

This Sufi meditation looks at the difference between what is and what we believe.

Mowlana Jalaluddin Rumi's story is as follows. A farmer went to his barn to check on a sick mule, and because it was dark, he did not see the lion asleep in the place of the mule who was then lying in another corner. The farmer put his hand out to stroke his mule and unknowingly stroked the shoulder of the lion. The farmer's heart was awakened.

If the farmer had seen what he was doing he would have been afraid. But because he was unafraid he received the lion's transmission of power. Rumi uses this story to explain the unseen power within us. Fearless exploration can reveal the roar within us.

If the farmer had been afraid, he would not have been able to absorb the lion's strength. This can be applied to speaking. Many people think that successful speakers have no fear, do not stutter; their hearts do not race, they can hear accurately, and they do not have stage fright. This isn't true. The same mechanisms are in play. Speakers stutter, famous actors stutter, but what is different is the fear of it. When a professional speaker stutters he continues because he has no fear of what it means. He is not embarrassed; he allows the power of the moment to emerge. Conversely, many famous actors and singers start developing anxiety by focusing on "What could happen if . . ."

Note: These meditations are practices for mental focus. The image of the farmer stroking the lion, thinking it to be his mule, and receiving the lion's strength is a good start. No one should do these mediations thinking that they can eliminate fear. The ability to see fear on one side and power on the other and be in the middle is the objective for all Raja meditations.

Hatha Yoga: Simhasana, the New Lion Pose

The Sanskrit word *simha,* which literally means "the powerful one," is the word for "lion." The posture Simhasana, therefore, is known as the Lion posture, and one performing it can be said to resemble a roaring lion about to attack. This position energizes and develops the physical mechanisms of speech. The Lion exercises form the cornerstone of the Yoga for Stuttering method. If you are unable to sit on the floor or cross your legs, you may sit on a chair.

Simhasana: Lion Pose

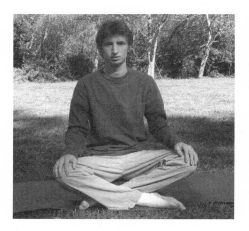

Sit with good posture, spine erect, cross-legged on the floor. Place your palms face down resting on your knees, stretching your fingers out as far as possible. Keep a straight back, neck, and shoulders.

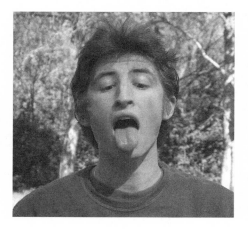

Breathe in through the nose, then open your mouth wide, sticking your tongue out as far as possible while looking at the tip of your nose or between your eyes and exhale, saying, "Ahhhhhhhhhhh." You can cross your eyes if you want (this is an additional movement that will improve your vision).

Inhale and expand your chest fully, imitating the lion. Without exhaling, slowly arch (hunch) your shoulders. Extend your throat and neck. Slowly open your mouth, lowering your chin as a lion would do to roar. Relax your throat and neck.

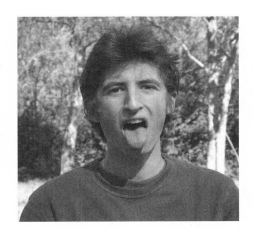

Remain in this breath-locking position for as long as you are comfortable.

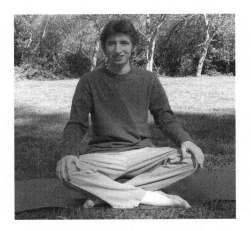

Nada Yoga: The Lion's Roar
While in the Lion pose, open your mouth as wide as possible; exhale and roar.

    RRRRROOOOOOOOOOAAAAAAAARRRRR

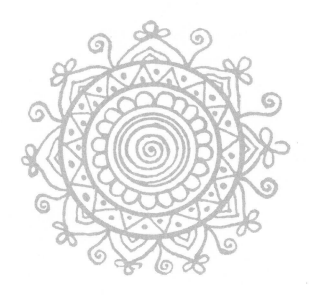

5

The Bee

Raja Yoga: The Saffron Bee

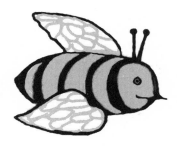

"With regular practice of this pranayama (Bhramari)
bliss arises in the yogi's heart."
—SWAMI SWATMARAMA

Bhramari refers to the Indian bumblebee. The exercise named after it primarily focuses on sounds and breath. *Bhramari* also describes the hum that is made and felt within the body during this exercise. The emphasis is on creating and feeling vibrations in the body.

In Sanskrit *bhramarin* means "that which produces ecstasy." The vibration of the *bhramari* is said to relax the brain. The Saffron Bee exercise combines *bhramari* with asanas that focus on hearing sound within the body.

The Egyptians considered bees to be the tears of the sun god, Ra. The temple of the goddess Neith is called "The House of the Bee." Honey symbolizes transformation through resurrection, and the bee, a protector from evil. Jars of honey were placed alongside Tutankhamen in his pyramid. The pharaohs were called "He of the Bee." *Bhramari*, like most transformative animals, may be feared. Simultaneously the bee is worshipped for its offerings. The Bhramari asana mimics the bee's vibration in order to obtain the bee's transformational quality.

Hatha Yoga: Bhramari, the Bee Exercise

There are successful musicians who cannot hear with their ears. Instead, they feel sound with other parts of their bodies. This exercise will help you feel the vibrations of vowels in the five parts of the body mentioned earlier: the crown, forehead, throat, chest, and gut.

Sit with a straight back. Place your hands on your knees. Inhale deeply through the nose and hold your breath.

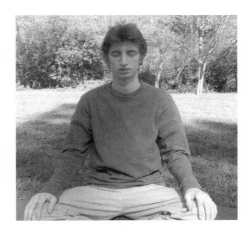

Raise your chin, relax your shoulders, and close your eyes.

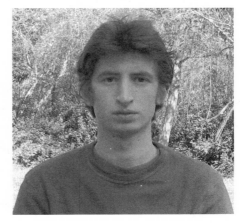

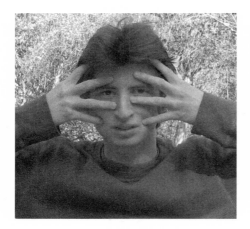

Make a mask with your fingers covering your eyes, using your thumbs to cover your ears.

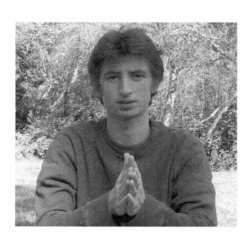

Make a smooth, deep, strong humming sound. Feel the vibrations in your whole body. After the exhalation, rub your hands together until they are warm.

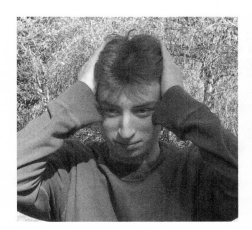 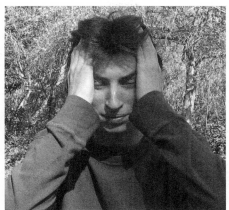

Move your palms up and over the face, then down to the neck, and back up over the cheeks, the forehead, and up to the crown.

Repeat this three to five times.

The goal is to feel the vibration of the bee's hum within the five parts of the body.

Nada Yoga: Humming Bee

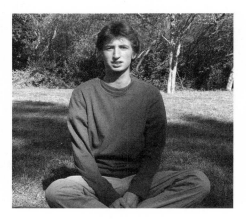

Using the Bhramari posture, produce a hum starting with "h" and ending with "e."

Hmmmmmmmmmmmmmmmm

Eeeeeeeeeeeeeeeeeeeeeeeeeeee

Using the above posture, produce a hum starting with "m" and ending with "e."

Mmmmmmmmmmmmmmmmm

Eeeeeeeeeeeeeeeeeeeeeeeeeeee

Using the above posture, produce a hum starting with "n" and ending with "e."

Nnnnnnnnnnnnnnnnnnnnnnnnn

Eeeeeeeeeeeeeeeeeeeeeeeeeee

Substitute the following and note the difference in vibrations, and where you feel them.

Hummmmmmmmmmmmmmm

Hommmmmmmmmmmmmmm

Himmmmmmmmmmmmmmm

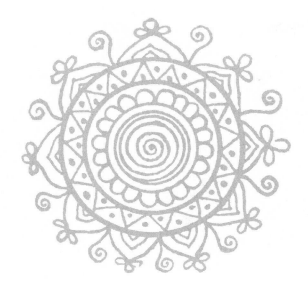

6

The Cobra

Raja Yoga: Snake

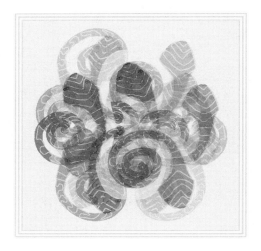

The snake has long been the symbol of healing. In fact, the American Medical Association uses the snake entwined with different Greek symbols in two of their logos. The first comes from the caduceus, the wand of Hermes, the messenger of the gods, and shows two snakes circling a wand. The second, the rod of Asclepius, the god of healing, shows one snake circling a rod. These symbols represent the healing arts by combining the snake, a symbol of rebirth and fertility, with a staff, a symbol of authority.

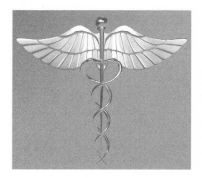 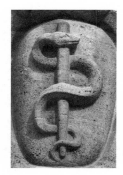

The Wand of Hermes and the Rod of Asclepius

In Hindu mythology, the cobra represents the cosmic power within us. One of the Hindu images of God, Shiva, wears a cobra around his neck or waist. When he dances as Nataraja, he represents the cosmos. Shiva's dance takes place in each of us at every level of our physical being. The birth of the world, its maintenance and destruction, and the soul's obscuration and liberation are the five acts of the dance.

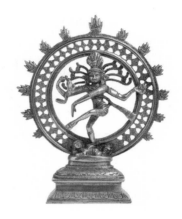

Image of Nataraja, the dancing form of the deity Shiva

In ancient Egypt, the goddess Wadjet took the form of a cobra to represent truth and justice. The cobra can also be seen on the top of the headdress of Egyptian pharaoh King Tutankhamun (King Tut). There, the rearing cobra, the uraeus, protects the Egyptians as they pass through the underworld.

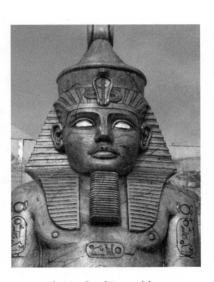

Death Mask of Tutankhamen

Another symbol of the snake's power is revealed in the story of Buddha's awakening. There was a horrible storm that threatened Buddha. A huge cobra rose above him to protect him from the storm. This is why the cobra's hood has finger marks; they are a blessing from Buddha.

In Christianity, although the snake could be seen as a symbol of evil in Genesis, Biblical historians point out that in the story of Adam and Eve, the snake also symbolizes transformation.... And Moses uses a snake to part the Red Sea and take the Jewish people to the promised land.

Bhujangasana is the name of the posture that represents the cobra's physical and mental focus.

Hatha Yoga: Bhujangasana, the Cobra Pose

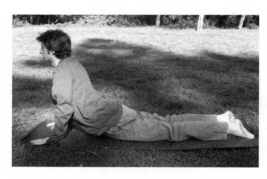

Lie on your stomach with your forehead on the floor with your palms slightly under your chest, your body in a straight line. Slowly inhale, then exhale as you lift your head and press your palms into the floor while raising your chest from your hips, keeping your legs flat on the floor. Remember, when you inhale, your stomach should expand, and when you exhale, your stomach should contract.

Hold this position breathing deeply and slowly for as long as you are comfortable. As you lower your body, exhale slowly and bring your arms to the sides of your body and relax.

Open your eyes wide as possible. Rapidly stick your tongue in and out as a snake would, darting your eyes left and right.

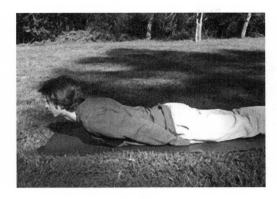

If you are feeling energetic, raise your upper body without using your hands.

If you do the advanced form on your stomach, coordinate your darting tongue with your breath. Your tongue should go out when your air goes out, and in when your breath comes in.

Start slowly, then increase to moderate and then rapid breathing. If you begin to hyperventilate, stop and just practice rapidly moving your tongue in and out, holding yourself upright on your hands.

Nada Yoga: Cobra

> *"The deer is entrapped by sweet sound. The cobra is enchanted by sweet music. Nada (sound) entraps the mind. The mind obtains bliss in sweet nada. Therefore you can easily control the mind through the practice of Nada Yoga."*
> —SWAMI SIVANANDA

Produce the "s" in the snake's hisssss clearly. "S" is an important phoneme because it is in eighty percent of all English words. If you are producing an unclear "s" you may sound sloppy and your speech may be unclear.

A simple way to produce "s" is to produce "t." With your tongue down keep the sides of the tongue on the teeth. The "s" sound should be sharp. It should not sound like "sh."

People who stutter may consider themselves disabled, but everyone has had the experience of being unable to speak clearly. I have been a competitive speaker and taught speech, yet two weeks ago when I found myself in front of an agent for this book I suddenly heard my "s" turn to "sh." I quickly practiced "t," "s," "t," "s." Anyone who uses her voice in performance will vocalize before going on stage. The Cobra exercise can help all kinds of speakers produce clear speech.

Not only is "s" in eighty percent of English words, it is also the sound that snakes produce: a powerful hiss. Using the visualization of the cobra's hiss winding around the body in a coil inside and out will produce a strong sense of sound, as well as develop the mechanical ability to prolong a very important phoneme in English.

In one breath start with the traditional "s" (snake hiss), taking it in and imagining it winding around your inside and then your outside.

Sssssssssssssssssssiiiiiiiiiiiiiiiiiiiii
Sssssssssssssssssssooooooooooooo
Sssssssssssssssssssaaaaaaaaaaaaaaa
Sssssssssssssssssssuuuuuuuuuuuuu

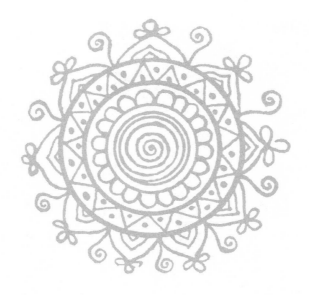

7

The Fish

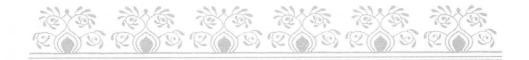

Raja Yoga: Transparent Fish

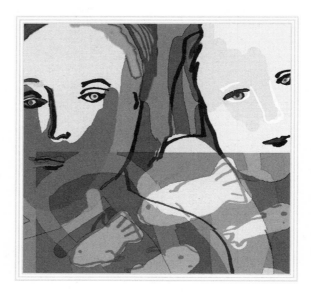

The fish symbolizes God's abundance. In Buddhism the fish has been said to signify fearlessness and happiness as it swims freely through the oceans without drowning. The sea in Buddhism is associated with the world of suffering, the cycle of samsara. The image of the golden fish is one of the eight auspicious symbols.

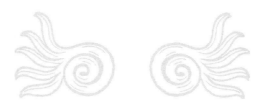

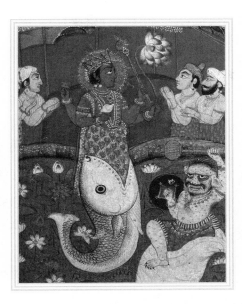

In his first incarnation, Lord Vishnu appeared as Matsya. Matsya has the torso of a man and the lower half of a fish. Vishnu assumed this form to save the world from the flood. In one of the stories of Matsya, the first king to rule the earth was washing his hands in a stream when a little fish swam into his hands and begged the king to save him. The benevolent king put the fish in a jar, which it soon outgrew. The king moved it first into a tank, then a river, and then the ocean. The fish then warned the king that a great flood would occur that would destroy all life. The fish revealed itself as Vishnu, and the king then built a boat that the fish towed to a mountaintop when the flood came. The king survived the flood, along with some "seeds of life" to reestablish life on earth.

This story shows us that in compassion we are blessed. The purpose of Yoga is to expand your consciousness. With incremental Yoga instruction—just as the fish grew—the power of your inner and outer voice will expand.

Hatha Yoga: Matyasana, and Other Fish Poses

Matsyasana: Fish pose

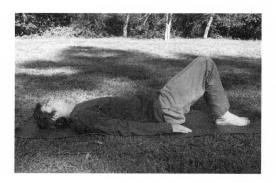

Lie on a smooth surface on your back, bend your knees, and put your hands at your sides.

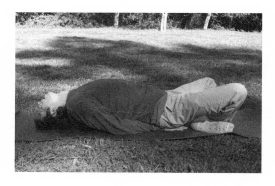

Arch your back, supported by your elbows if necessary. Lean backwards, resting the crown of your head on the floor.

Use your forearms and elbows to support you as you expand your chest. Breathe deeply.

Remain in this asana for about one minute.

Matsyendrasana: Lord of the Fishes Pose

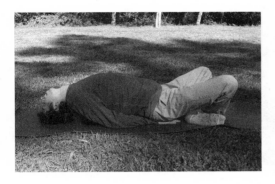 Lie on your back with your knees bent, feet on the floor. Inhale, lift your pelvis slightly off the floor, and slide your hands, palms down, below your buttocks.

Then rest your buttocks on the backs of your hands (don't lift off your hands as you perform this pose). Put your arms close to your sides. Inhale and press your forearms and elbows firmly against the floor.

Next press your scapulas into your back and, with an inhale, lift your upper torso and head away from the floor. Squeeze the thigh muscles up toward the belly.

Ardha Matsyendrasana: Half Lord of the Fishes Pose

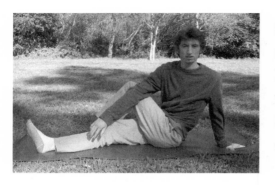

Sit on the floor with your legs straight out in front of you. Bend your left knee and cross your left foot over your right leg. The right knee points directly up at the ceiling.

Exhale and twist toward the inside of the left thigh.

Press the inner left foot very actively into the floor, release the groin, and lengthen the front torso. Lean back slightly, against the shoulder blades, and continue to lengthen the back, supported by the floor.

With every inhalation, lift a little more through the sternum, pushing the fingers against the floor to help.

Switch legs, and repeat the position on the opposite side.

Nada Yoga: Transparent Fish

You can sit down or lie down to do this exercise.

Take a long, slow, deep breath through your nose.

Close the throat by holding your neck muscles and lower jaw tense.

Breathe in, expanding your chest, and as you exhale through your mouth, produce a deep "shh" sound with the teeth together, similar to the sound of the ocean. Lengthen the inhalation and the exhalation as much as possible without creating tension anywhere in your body, and allow the sound of the breath to be continuous and smooth.

Tip: To help create the proper "ah" sound, hold your hand up to your mouth and exhale as if trying to fog a mirror. Inhale the same way. Notice how you constrict the back of the throat to create the fog effect. Now close your mouth and do the same thing while breathing through the nose.

8

The Wolf

Raja Yoga: Native American Wolf

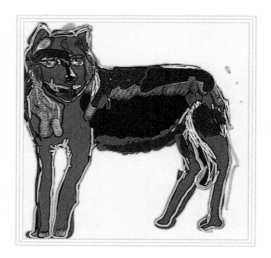

The wolf, considered a symbol of strength by Native Americans, represents a solitary path, perhaps because wolves, unlike other wild dogs, often travel alone. To truly come to understand oneself, one must be able to be alone, undistracted by, nor dependent on, the opinions of others. One must learn to listen to the voice within, which—in silence—speaks as clearly as the sound of a wolf howling in the night. This posture is about taking a full breath and exhaling while producing a howl.

Hatha Yoga: Native American Wolf

Get on your hands and knees with a straight back. Straighten your arms. Sit back onto your feet.

Go back to the position on your hands and knees. Expand your chest, lean your head back, and howl with a long stream of breath.

Nada Yoga: Native American Wolf

The Wolf asana is an introduction to overtoning. Overtoning occurs when two vowel sounds are made simultaneously. The harmonics are produced because of the vibration. When it is done properly it is very exciting because the listener may have trouble distinguishing what sounds the singer is producing—but the singer knows.

Create wolf howls in any variation or combination of the "ou" and "ooo" sounds:

Owwwwwwwwwooooooooooooo

Produce as long a howl as you can, and record the length of time.

9

The Grasshopper

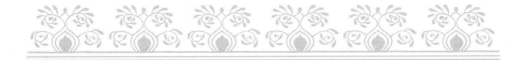

Raja Yoga: Grasshopper

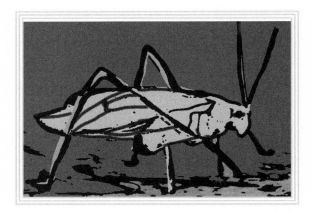

In Asia, the grasshopper is a symbol of good luck. The grasshopper represents an abundance of energy contained in a small vessel. The amazing grasshopper can fly through the air by springing with its tiny legs that appear to be made of material lighter than straw.

En masse, they are called locusts. They descend on crops, devouring and destroying everything, defined in the Bible as a plague. In Proverbs 30:27, they are presented as an example of the strength of unity: "The locusts have no king, yet they all advance in ranks."

Together humans can provide for each other, and as a group, we can protect each other from danger. We learn from the research and experience of other humans. Yoga traditions, established thousands of years ago, help us now. As you practice this posture, reflect on the support inherent in being part of a group.

Hatha Yoga: Shalabhasana, the Grasshopper Pose

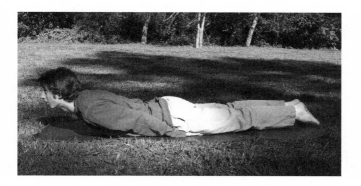

Lie on your stomach with your head turned to one side and your arms alongside your body with palms facing upward. Place your chin on the floor. Slide your hands under your thighs, with the palms pressed gently against the top of your thighs.

Inhale slowly, then, as you exhale, raise your head and chest off the floor as high as possible. Tilt your head as far back as possible. Keep your feet, knees, and thighs pressed together.

Starting at the top of your head and working your way down to your feet, bring your attention to each part of your body, consciously relaxing it before proceeding on to the next.

Hold the posture for as long as you can hold your inhaled breath, then exhale and slowly return your chest and head to the floor. Place your arms beside your body.

Nada Yoga: Grasshopper

This exercise provides skill in putting consonants with prolonged vowels. The grasshopper's click is a sound that develops our tongue coordination.

Voooooooooooooooooooooooooooooooom

Viiiiiiiiiiiiiiiiiiiiiiiiiiiiiiiiiiiiiiiiiiiiiim

Huuuuuuuuuuuuuuuuuuuuuuuuuuuuuuuuum

Hiiiiiiiiiiiiiiiiiiiiiiiiiiiiiiiiiiiiiiiiiiiiiiii

Listen to the actual sounds of grasshoppers, which are very gentle, and pick your own sounds to imitate. The emphasis is on one prolonged sound.

10

The Elephant

Raja Yoga: Elephant

The Precious Elephant, Sri Ganapati

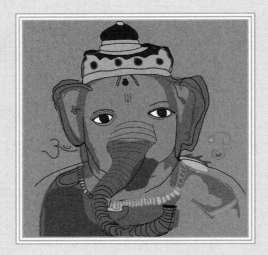

Ganesh is the elephant-headed son of the deities Shiva and Parvati. He is a much-loved deity in India, where he is considered the remover of obstacles; the elephant can demolish most things because of its size and strength. Ganesh is invoked at the beginning of all important ventures to ensure success, such as in marriage ceremonies to ensure a trouble-free relationship for the bride and groom. In his dancing form, Ganesh is called Ganapati.

Hatha Yoga: Ganapati Asana

In India, the swaying gait and the slow, elegant movements of the elephant are considered the epitome of power and gracefulness. The elephant's movements are gentle, but a herd of them can destroy a town. The elephant is also associated with the earth and its tremors. The ground is said to tremble as the herds pass. According to one regional myth, the world rests on the head of a great elephant, Mahapadma, and earthquakes are produced when it moves its head to get more comfortable.

Stand upright.

Drop your chin to your chest.

With tension applied to the neck muscles and a slow inhalation through your nose, pull your head up slowly and gently until the forehead looks upward to the ceiling.

Drop the head with a quick exhalation through the nose so that the chin strikes the chest gently with a bounce.

Perform this technique daily: six times in the morning and six times in the evening.

You can also practice pranayama while performing this asana. The three sequences described below should be performed in the morning and evening, and can be repeated several times. For further pranayama practice, use the resources in the back of this book to find a qualified teacher.

Sit in the asana for pranayama with your back straight, eyes closed, and chin parallel to the floor.

Drop your chin to your chest and puff your chest out with a curve to your spine. With your eyes closed, breathe in through your nose with your mouth closed, pulling the air into your breastbone.

By partially closing the back of your throat, make a sobbing noise while inhaling, feeling the cool air against the palate.

Hold the air in your upper chest for six seconds, feeling the expansion of the chest.

Exhale slowly through your nose, creating a sobbing sound, feeling a warm current of air on the palate. Both inhalation and exhalation should take from ten to twelve seconds.

Perform sixteen such breaths in the morning and sixteen in the evening.

After the above technique is practiced, remain in the asana of pranayama for several minutes in silence, preparing for the following technique.

Open your mouth and stick your tongue out slightly, curling your tongue to create a tube through which to breathe. If you are unable to curl your tongue, slightly tense your lips to create the "tube" and simply touch your lower lip with your tongue. The breathing should be cooling to your lips, tongue, and system.

With a slow inhalation, fill your lower lungs completely with deep diaphragmatic breathing, then fill your upper lungs.

Remain in the asana of pranayama and prepare to perform *Nadi Shodhana,* the last technique.

Nada Yoga: Obstacle Remover

Nadi Shodhana is a method of alternate nostril breathing suitable for beginners and advanced students. *Nadi* refers to the energy pathways through which *prana* flows. Nadi Shodhana means "channel cleaning." It calms the mind, soothes anxiety and stress, balances left and right hemispheres, and promotes clear thinking.

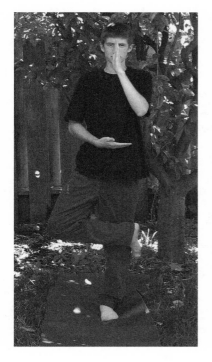

Hold your right hand up and curl your index and middle fingers toward your palm. Place your thumb next to your right nostril and your ring finger and pinky by your left nostril. Close your right nostril by pressing gently against it with your thumb, and inhale through your left nostril. The breath should be slow, steady, and full.

Now close your left nostril by pressing gently against it with your ring finger and pinky, open your right nostril by relaxing your thumb, and exhale fully with a slow and steady breath.

Inhale through your right nostril, close it, and then exhale through your left nostril.

Inhale through the left; exhale through the right.

Inhale through the right; exhale through the left.

Begin with five to ten rounds and add more as you feel ready. Remember to keep your breathing slow, easy, and full.

You can do this as part of your centering before beginning an asana or posture routine, or at different times throughout the day. Nadi Shodhana helps control stress and anxiety. If you start to feel stressed, ten or so rounds will help calm you down. It also helps soothe anxiety caused by flying or other fearful or stressful situations.

This is a nice chant:

Om Ganapati Namo Nama Om Ganapati Namo Nama

Produce the following groups slowly.

Gum, Gome, Gim, Gam
Roam, Rum, Rim, Ran
Hey, Ho, Ha, Hay, He, Ho

The Hoop

Imagine the sound "o" as a vibrational Hula-hoop, coming out of you and surrounding you, going around and around.

The Ladder

Think of the letter A. It looks like a ladder. Imagine that ladder is very long. Start by saying the vowel A on as low a note as you can manage, and go up the scale step by step on **one** breath. This exercise is similar to singing scales. Try this with the other vowels once you have mastered the A. Be aware of the vowel or the range of notes your body feels most comfortable with.

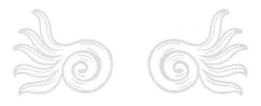

11

The Peacock

Raja Yoga: Peacock Feathers Down

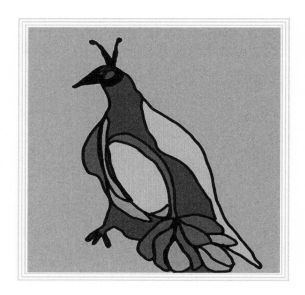

In the South Asian myth of creation, the universe was created from a sea of milk. Within this sea of milk was a primordial poison. The peacock swallows the poison and transforms it into immortality. The peacock symbolizes victory over poisonous tendencies in humans. It is a symbol of transformation.

Hatha Yoga: The White Peacock

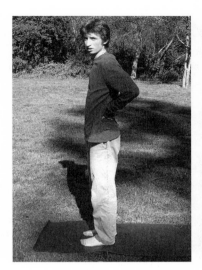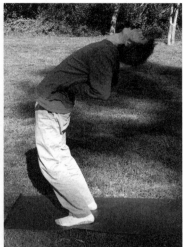

The Peacock: Mayurasana

This asana is a variation of the Peacock posture. Start in a standing position, put your hands on your lower back, and slowly bend backward. Breath deeply.

Nada Yoga: Peacock

When we stutter, we are out of synch. Our brain is sending a message to our bodies, but the vocal mechanism is moving out of synch with our intentions. To increase the agility of your vocal mechanism—your mouth—you can use standard tongue twisters. The first one is the most important. Start slow and speed up. If you have a friend who will sing with you (kids like to do these exercises) have them do it with you because you can hear overtones (harmonics) that occur because of the juxtaposition of vibrations.

Say the following slowly and repeat, speeding up each time.

Ring, Rang, Rung, Rong

Sing, Sang, Sung, Song

Round and round the rugged rock the ragged rascal ran.

Case Study: Alex—Expanding Time

Alex was a very successful businessman. He looked a bit like George Carlin and was a very devout person; he would observe silence and didn't speak at all one day of the week. He only found his stuttering take over when he was excited. His personality too was a bit like George Carlin's. He couldn't figure out what made him stutter. He liked to move rapidly, and when he was moving rapidly he didn't stutter. He came to see me and was in a very distressed mood. He was getting a divorce and his stuttering had become overwhelming. He was worried about bringing in an income since he was self-employed, and he was beginning to panic about getting clients.

Speaking to Alex, I realized that he never stopped weighing the possibilities of doom and trying to prepare for what he didn't know. Since he couldn't work out all the possibilities, his mind stuttered; his voice was just a by-product. He spoke faster and faster until his mind had to pause his speech, like a CD that gets stuck because too much information is being processed. Through the Yoga for Stuttering exercises and meditations, Alex learned how to produce a very slow utterance, which enabled him to slow his thoughts down to a manageable speed and subsequently improve his fluency and ability to communicate.

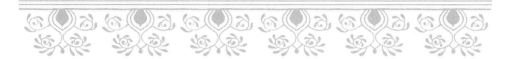

Afterword

This book is the culmination of ten years of work. Each year I have found more studies to strengthen my understanding of why using prolonged sounds helps stuttering. It has been difficult to distill all that I have learned into these basic lessons; however, they are effective and powerful, and I hope that I have presented them in a manner that can be easily used.

It has been rewarding as a speech therapist and as a researcher to read about the work in Yoga and neurology. International research is ongoing, and I seem to find more material each day that I would like to include in this book. Yoga for Stuttering is just the beginning. The core of this method is to develop the capacity to produce long, strong sounds necessary for speaking and singing. It is my hope that all Yoga for Stuttering students will find themselves interested in the continued development of their voices beyond overcoming disfluency. The potential of the human voice is rarely tapped.

Recently I heard an opera singer singing in a shopping center at a fundraising event. She had no amplification, but you could hear her three or four blocks away. Her singing was a truly amazing demonstration of the power and strength of the human voice. It occurred to me then that operatic vocal training is founded on prolonged utterances, and that perhaps the exercises practiced by opera singers have a great deal in common with the

Yoga for Stuttering exercises presented in this book. Vocal exercises, performed with the correct attitude of relaxation, have the effect of invigorating the energy centers of the body, bringing together the body and mind to produce a harmonious state of being.

Stuttering is only one type of speech disorder that can be improved through this method. I encourage you to be creative with your voice. This is the beginning of a new road. Hopefully you will get as much pleasure from practicing this program as I have had teaching it, and I wish you the best on your path.

Resources

This book is for those who want to work independently; however, the American Speech-Language-Hearing Association can help you find an individual speech therapist should you need support in working through this program. There are numerous Yoga associations in the United States that can direct you to classes and teachers; try Yoga Finder and Yoga Alliance, listed below. If you find the Raja Yoga portions of this program to be effective, there are many meditation centers around the world that provide programs.

Here is a list of Web sites and organizations that help people find yoga classes, speech therapists, etc.

American Yoga Association: www.americanyogaassociation.org

American Speech-Language-Hearing Association: www.asha.org

Spirit Rock Meditation Center: www.spiritrock.org

Yoga Alliance: www.yogaalliance.org

Yoga Finder: www.yogafinder.com

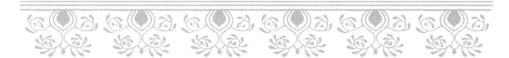

Recommended Reading

Abitbol, Jean. *Odyssey of the Voice*. San Diego, CA: Plural Publishing, 2006.

> This book is excellently written by a French oncologist. It conveys scientific analysis and lays out in fascinating detail the psychology of voice and its emotional effects on the body.

Andrews, Ted. *Sacred Sounds: Magic and Healing through Words and Music*. St. Paul: Llewellyn, 1992.

> This book deals with the chakras and how they are affected by sound. The author shows what notes heal each part of the body, and how you can use tuning forks to feel the sounds. He suggests having groups sing while each person lies in a different geometrical shape, and then comparing results. He explains how shapes promote the sound to intensify transformation. I have tried this fun exercise with groups of students and found it interesting to share how we each experienced it.

Bennett, Bija. *Emotional Yoga: How the Body Can Heal the Mind*. New York: Simon & Schuster, 2002.

> This book has developed a set of postures aimed at healing emotional states. The asanas are based on the standard, but adapted for the Western person who is concerned about specific emotional issues. Since stuttering has an emotional component, this book is a good way to lead into pranayama. A good introduction for the Western mind.

Bobrick, Benson. *Knotted Tongues: Stuttering in History and the Quest for a Cure.* New York: Simon & Schuster, 1995.

Bobrick, who grew up stuttering severely, writes a compelling book about the history of stuttering and the different, sometimes horrific, historical cures. He also provides a history of stuttering (including the fact that Moses stuttered). Bobrick found a program that helped him considerably, and he has not stuttered since.

Campbell, Don G. *Music: Physician for Times to Come.* Wheaton, IL: Quest Books, 2007.

This is an excellent book that provides essays by those working in the music-as-healing field, including musicians, medical doctors, and alternative healers. The basis of this work is that music has always been used to change emotional states, and that the sound of the human voice evokes different physical responses in the body and brain.

———. *The Roar of Silence: Healing Powers of Breath, Tone and Music.* Wheaton, IL: Theosophical Publishing House with assistance from the Kern Foundation, 1989.

The book is the story of the author, who was healed by music.

Carter, Rita, and Christopher D. Frith. *Mapping the Mind.* Berkeley: University of California Press, 1998.

This book is fascinating. Page 155 shows both the right and left hemispheres of the brain of a person who stutters. Discussion of the brain functions is put in language that someone new to neurology can easily understand. The book has great illustrations and interesting facts about the human brain.

Chapman, Jessie. *Yoga Therapies*. Berkeley, CA: Ulysses Press, 2003.

> This is an illustrated book of Yoga asanas laid out in forty sequences. You have to hunt for the postures that would help with specific problems, including sports injuries, headaches, weight issues, etc. It's full of photos and includes an ample index.

Choudhury, Bikram, and Bonnie Jones Reynolds. *Bikram's Beginning Yoga Class*. New York: Jeremy P. Tarcher/Putnam, 2000.

> I got into Yoga because there was a Bikram studio around the corner from my house. Bikram Yoga has twenty-six postures that take an hour and a half and are done at a room temperature of approximately 100–125 degrees Fahrenheit. It's fun, but rather intensive.

Coulter, H. David. *Anatomy of Hatha Yoga: A Manual for Students, Teachers, and Practitioners*. Honesdale, PA: Body Breath, 2001.

> This book is 621 pages of detailed anatomy of asanas. It's an excellent reference, and would benefit Yoga teachers as well as those who need to identify specific ligaments in a posture.

D'Angelo, James. *The Healing Power of the Human Voice: Mantras, Chants, and Seed Sounds for Health and Harmony*. Rochester, VT: Healing Arts Press, 2005.

> The author is from the United Kingdom. He provides information about European sound healing societies. He has included specific sounds for body organs and provides an extensive list of organizations throughout the world that have conferences and workshops.

Dewhurst-Maddock, Olivea. *The Book of Sound Therapy: Heal Yourself with Music and Voice*. New York: Simon & Schuster, 1993.

> This is a very nice coffee-table book to review the different aspects of sound therapy. Photos and pictures throughout.

Easwaran, Eknath. *The Mantram Handbook*. Tomales, CA: Nilgiri Press, 2001.

> All phonemes are technically mantras: units of pure sound. *Mantram* are units of sound associated with aspects of the universe. Although this is a small book it has a lot of information. The author reveals that sounds heard in the heart are our own resonance with the universe. Hearing a pure sound, with intention, manifests permanent peace.

Gardner, Kay. *Sounding the Inner Landscape*. Rockport, MA: Element Books, 1990.

> The author is a musician and has a large section that relates music to different parts of the body. She emphasizes finding our own music that is authentic to our self—this music will heal us.

Garfield, Laeh Maggie. *Sound Medicine: Healing with Music, Voice, and Song*. Berkeley, CA: Celestial Arts, 1987.

> This book provides discussion of alternative ways at looking at sound healing.

Gass, Robert, and Kathleen Brehony. *Chanting: Discovering Spirit in Sound*. New York: Broadway Books, 1999.

> This book is great. After attending Harvard, Robert Gass, a musician and clinical psychologist, found himself attracted to chanting and here provides a volume of material on the subject. Well thought out, and easy to use. The authors have collected chants from around the world and explain the significance behind them. Gass feels that chanting is important because of the ritual and because of the positive effect of sound on the body. He has also recorded a whole line of music based on chanting. This book also provides good references to chanting groups.

Gaynor, Mitchell L., MD. *Sounds of Healing: A Physician Reveals the Therapeutic Power of Sound, Voice, and Music.* New York: Broadway Books, 1999.

> Dr. Gaynor is an oncologist who uses sounds with cancer patients. He explains his techniques using sound in the healing process, and asserts that sound can be preventive as well. The book gives good incentive to sing, chant, and play an instrument.

Godwin, Joscelyn. *The Mystery of the Seven Vowels: In Theory and Practice.* Grand Rapids, MI: Phanes Press, 1991.

> An in-depth discussion on the historical use of vowels as sacred sounds.

Goldman, Jonathan. *Healing Sounds: The Power of Harmonics.* Shaftesbury, Dorset: Element Books, 1992.

> Excellent discussion on the author's own discovery of overtones.

Iyengar, B. K. S. *Light on Pranayama: The Yogic Art of Breathing.* New York: Crossroad Publishing Co., 1985.

———. *Light on Yoga.* New York: Schocken Books, 1995.

> These books are the classics for American readers. When I started Yoga at UC Berkeley in 1975, my teacher, "Sunny," required *Light on Yoga.* At that time, the teaching style was very fierce, and right after the class I threw the book into the garbage. I think I have bought the book several times since then. Iyengar was one of the first to catalog the asanas that emerged from different teachers.

Kadetsky, Elizabeth. *First There Is a Mountain: A Yoga Romance.* Boston: Little, Brown & Co., 2004.

> I included this book because I enjoy first-person perspective. Kadetsky is a writer who finds that her health is crumbling. This is

the story of her travel to study with Iyengar. She comes with her own problems (she has an eating disorder) but she doesn't dwell on them. She provides quite a bit of information on Iyengar, his method, and her experiences at his institute in India. One interesting point she makes is that we have more Yoga studios in California than in all of India, and India is a very big place. Yoga is a throwback, an ancient tradition that the West has adopted and practiced but that is largely forgotten by its country of origin.

Kaminoff, Leslie, Amy Matthews, and Sharon Ellis. *Yoga Anatomy.* Chicago: Human Kinetics, 2007.

This is one of my favorite books. It provides a clear illustration of each asana and the muscles involved, which I'm especially interested in as a speech pathologist. For instance, if you like a specific posture, you can see exactly what muscles are affected and pick postures that target specific muscles.

Khalsa, Guru Dharam Singh, and Darryl O'Keeffe. *The Kundalini Yoga Experience: Bringing Body, Mind, and Spirit Together.* New York: Simon & Schuster, 2002.

These are very well laid-out Yoga exercises. Of the Hatha Yoga forms in the United States, Kundalini Yoga is the most focused on the breath.

Mehta, Silva, Mira Mehta, and Shyam Mehta. *Yoga: The Iyengar Way; The New Definitive Guide to the Most Practised Form of Yoga.* New York: Alfred A. Knopf, 1990.

This book has photos, and a lot of them. It is a very good book to do Yoga with since you can see each side of the asana.

Parry, William D. *Understanding and Controlling Stuttering: A Comprehensive New Approach Based on the Valsalva Hypothesis.* Anaheim Hills, CA: National Stuttering Association, 2000.

> The National Stuttering Association distributes this and many other books and resources. This book stands out as proposing a new therapy based on prolonged breath. I included it because Parry clearly explains the mechanisms of stuttering and speech.

Paul, Russill. *The Yoga of Sound: Healing and Enlightenment through the Sacred Practice of Mantra.* Novato, CA: New World Library, 2004.

> Paul's extensive book explains all of the different forms of Yoga and their practices. He is also a musician and has included a CD. A good book for a beginner in the study of Yoga.

Penfield, Wilder, and Lamar Roberts. *Speech and Brain Mechanisms.* Princeton, NJ: Princeton University Press, 1959.

> This is an excellent book on speech anatomy. It gives solid information for the layperson but also goes into depth. Includes actual photos of the brain.

Perlmutter, Leonard, and Jenness Cortez Perlmutter. *The Heart and Science of Yoga: A Blueprint for Peace, Happiness and Freedom from Fear.* New York: AMI Publishers, 2005.

> This is an excellent book with a comprehensive look at a beginner level for the Western reader. The authors cover each area of Yoga in clear language. They include references, personal anecdotes, and beginning exercises. This book goes into depth and yet is very accessible. If you're interested in Hatha Yoga, I recommend this book in addition to taking a class.

Radha, Swami Sivananda. *Mantras: Words of Power.* Spokane, WA: Timeless Books, 1994.

> Swami Radha was a well-known European dancer who went to India and met her guru, who told her to go back to the West and teach. She started an ashram and continued her Yoga lineage. She writes very well, and explains mantras from a historical perspective. She includes examples of her students who used mantras to work through psychological issues.

Rama, Swami. *Path of Fire and Light.* Vol. 1, *Advanced Practices of Yoga.* Honesdale, PA: Himalayan Institute Press, 1986.

> This is a very in-depth explanation and instruction for pranayama. Swami Rama also explores diet. This book is very well thought out and designed so as not to overwhelm you. Swami Rama says it is best to have a conservative approach, doing only what feels comfortable until it becomes easy.

Rama, Swami, Rudolph Ballentine, MD, and Alan Hymes, MD. *Science of Breath: A Practical Guide.* Honesdale, PA: Himalayan Institute Press, 1998.

> Swami Rama provides an excellent written explanation of pranayama.

Robin, Mel. *A Physiological Handbook for Teachers of Yogasana.* Tucson: Fenestra Books, 2002.

> This is the best overview of Yoga asanas I have seen. Robin goes into detail about why the asanas work. He provides a great index so that you can easily find the best postures for your specific ailment.

Rosen, Richard. *Pranayama: Beyond the Fundamentals.* Boston: Shambhala Publications, 2006.

————. *The Yoga of Breath: A Step-by-Step Guide to Pranayama.* Boston: Shambhala Publications, 2002.

> Pranayama is a complete Yoga in itself with strong traditions. The rule of thumb has always been: Don't do it without a teacher. On the surface, controlling your breath by breathing in specific ways seems uneventful; however, every time I read the warnings that attempting pranayama without supervision could cause anxiety and other problems, I back off. An interesting note is that one woman from Brooklyn used pranayama to lose weight, and subsequently became a guru. Rosen's book is especially interesting because he includes his own experience. He believes that blocks in energy can be worked through using his pranayama techniques. The book is very informative and simple to follow. Rosen also teaches Yoga and is accessible via the Web.

Shear, Jonathan, ed. *The Experience of Meditation: Experts Introduce the Major Traditions.* St. Paul: Paragon House, 2006.

> This is a good general introduction to meditation.

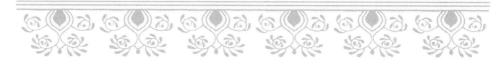

Glossary

aum, ohm, om. A mantra that represents both the unmanifest and manifest aspects of God.

aphasia. A loss of the ability to produce and/or comprehend language, due to injury to the brain areas that control speech functions: Broca's area, which governs language production, or Wernicke's area, which governs the interpretation of language.

apraxia. A neurological disorder characterized by loss of the ability to execute or carry out learned, purposeful movements, despite having the desire and the physical ability to perform the movements.

asana. A Sanskrit word meaning "seat" or "pose."

Bhagavad Gita. Lord Krishna's sermon to Arjuna in the *Mahabharata* epic, which consists of seven hundred verses.

bhramari. The Sanskrit word for the black Indian bumblebee.

bhramarin. A Sanskrit word meaning "sweet as honey" or "that which produces ecstasy."

Bhujangasana. The Cobra pose

diphthong. A sound composed of two vowel elements joined to form one sound.

disfluency. A break or interruption in otherwise normal speech.

Ganapati asana. The Elephant pose

Ganesh, Ganesha. The elephant-headed son of the deities Shiva and Parvati, worshiped as the remover of obstacles.

Hatha Yoga. The Yoga of movement. The word *hatha* comes from the Sanskrit terms *ha,* meaning "sun," and *tha,* meaning "moon." Hatha Yoga is union through movement.

hyper-focus. An intense form of mental concentration or visualization that focuses consciousness on a narrow subject, or beyond objective reality and onto subjective mental planes, daydreams, concepts, fiction, the imagination, and other objects of the mind. The ability to focus intently.

Matsyasana. The Fish pose

Matsyendrasana. Lord of the Fishes poses

Mayurasana. The Peacock pose

Melodic Intonation Therapy. A method that uses melodic and rhythmic components to stimulate activity in the right hemisphere of the brain in order to assist in speech production.

Nada Yoga. The Yoga of sound. Nada Yoga is a way of tapping into a stream of sacred sound that incorporates the full spectrum of frequencies—both those that are audible to the human ear and those that are inaudible. This means that all forms of music, the sounds of space, and even the entire electromagnetic spectrum of frequencies are included within this range of perception.

overtoning. A powerful healing modality involving using the voice to make more than one sound at a time.

phoneme. A single unit of sound in a language, for example "t" or "sh."

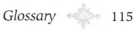

prana. The Sanskrit word for "breath"; the notion of a vital, life-sustaining force.

pranayama. A Sanskrit word meaning "lengthening of the prana or breath." It is often translated as "control of the life force." When used in Yoga, it is often translated as "breath control."

Raja Yoga. The form of Yoga that is most concerned with the cultivation of the mind using meditation.

samsara. A Sanskrit term for "continuous movement" or "continuous flowing." In Buddhism, samsara refers to the concept of a cycle of birth and consequent decay and death, in which all beings in the universe participate and which can be escaped only through enlightenment.

Shalabhasana. The Grasshopper pose.

simha. The Sanskrit word meaning "the powerful one"; also the word for "lion."

Simhasana. The Lion pose.

selective mutism. Typically a symptom of an anxiety disorder in which a person who is normally capable of speech is unable to speak in given situations, or to specific people. People with the disorder are fully capable of speech and understanding language, but can fail to speak in certain social situations when it is expected of them. Other symptoms associated with selective mutism can include excessive shyness, withdrawal, dependency upon parents, and oppositional behavior. Most cases of selective mutism are not the result of a single traumatic event, but rather are the manifestation of a chronic pattern of anxiety.

Sri Lalita Sahasranama. A twelfth-century Indian sutra composed of one thousand individual mantras describing various aspects of the Divine Mother.

Notes

1. Laeh Maggie Garfield, *Sound Medicine: Healing with Music, Voice, and Song* (Berkeley, CA: Celestial Arts, 1987).

2. Mitchell L. Gaynor, MD, *Sounds of Healing: A Physician Reveals the Therapeutic Power of Sound, Voice, and Music* (New York: Broadway Books, 1999).

3. Peter Fox, "Brain Imaging and Stuttering," *Journal of Fluency Disorders* 28, no. 4 (2003): 265–72.

4. Nicki S. Cohen, "The Effect of Singing Instruction on the Speech Production of Neurologically Impaired Persons," *Journal of Music Therapy* 29, no. 2 (1992): 87–100.

5. P. Belin et al., "Recovery from Nonfluent Aphasia after Melodic Intonation Therapy: A PET Study," *Neurology* 47:1504–11.

6. E. Yairi and N. Ambrose, "Stuttering: Recent Developments and Future Directions," *ASHA Leader,* 2004, 4–5, 14–15.

7. Benson Bobrick, *Knotted Tongues: Stuttering in History and the Quest for a Cure* (New York: Simon & Schuster, 1995).

8. M. L. Albert, R. W. Sparks, and N. A. Helm, "Melodic Intonation Therapy for Aphasia," *Archives for Neurology* 29 (1973): 130–31.

9. Noel Marshall and Pat Holtzapple, "Melodic Intonation Therapy: Variations on a Theme," in *Clinical Aphasiology Conference: 6th: Wemme, OR: May 18–21, 1976,* ed. Robert H. Brookshire (Minneapolis: BRK Publishers, 1976): 115–41.

10. J. C. Stemple, J. Stanley, and L. Lee, "Objective Measures of Voice Production in Normal Subjects Following Prolonged Voice Use," *Journal of Voice* 9 (1995): 127–33.

11. Mark Onslow, Janis Van Doorn, and Denis Newman, "Variability of Acoustic Segment Durations after Prolonged-Speech Treatment for Stuttering," *Journal of Speech and Hearing Research* 35 (June 1992): 529–36.

12. Swami Adiswarananda, *The Four Yogas: A Guide to the Spiritual Paths of Action, Devotion, Meditation, and Knowledge* (New York: Skylight Paths Publishing, 2006).

13. Russill Paul, *The Yoga of Sound: Healing and Enlightenment through the Sacred Practice of Mantra* (Novato, CA: New World Library, 2004).

14. Jonathan Shear, ed., *The Experience of Meditation: Experts Introduce the Major Traditions* (St. Paul: Paragon House, 2006).

15. Janice Chapman, *Singing and Teaching Singing: A Holistic Approach to Classical Voice* (San Diego, CA: Plural Publishing, 2006).

16. K. Uma et al., "The Integrated Approach of Yoga: A Therapeutic Tool for Mentally Retarded Children: A One-year Controlled Study," *Journal of Mental Deficiency Research* 33 (1989): 415–21.

17. Jean Abitbol, *Odyssey of the Voice* (San Diego, CA: Plural Publishing, 2006).

18. Bija Bennett, *Emotional Yoga: How the Body Can Heal the Mind* (New York: Simon & Schuster, 2002).

19. Richard Rosen, *The Yoga of Breath: A Step-by-Step Guide to Pranayama* (Boston: Shambhala Publications, 2002).

20. For a full discussion of the uses of chants, see Robert Gass and Kathleen Brehony, *Chanting: Discovering Spirit in Sound* (New York: Broadway Books, 1999); Ted Andrews, *Sacred Sounds: Magic and Healing through Words and Music* (St. Paul: Llewellyn, 1992); and Swami Sivananda Radha, *Mantras: Words of Power* (Spokane, WA: Timeless Books, 1994).

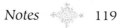

21. Olivea Dewhurst-Maddock, *The Book of Sound Therapy: Heal Yourself with Music and Voice* (New York: Simon & Schuster, 1993).

22. Cohen, "Effect of Singing Instruction."

23. Leslie Kaminoff, Amy Matthews, and Sharon Ellis, *Yoga Anatomy* (Chicago: Human Kinetics, 2007).

24. Swami Rama, Rudolph Ballentine, MD, and Alan Hymes, MD, *Science of Breath: A Practical Guide* (Honesdale, PA: Himalayan Institute Press, 1998).

25. R. Schum, "Clinical Perspectives on the Treatment of Selective Mutism," *Journal of Speech-Language Pathology and Applied Behavior Analysis* 1, no. 2 (2006): 149–63.

26. Dilgo Khyentse, "Like a Mirror, Like a Rainbow, Like the Heart of the Sun," *The Best Buddhist Writing 2004,* ed. Melvin Mcleod (Boston: Shambhala Publications, 2004): 183–95.

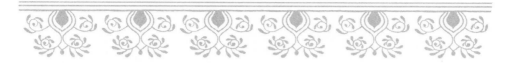

Index

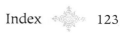

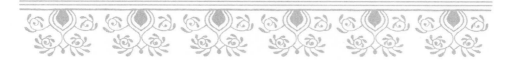

Acknowledgments

I am most grateful to all my speech students who have inspired me to be creative in my approach to their challenges. Their perseverance compelled me to explore, and share, this method. Thanks to my husband, David Balakrishnan, for listening to me and helping me understand Vedic philosophy, and to my son, Sam Mansfield, for allowing me to include him in the book, and for keeping my cup full of exquisitely prepared tea. I am indebted to my editor, Hisae Matsuda, for her guidance, support, and encouragement, and to my Sanskrit teacher, Ramana Erickson, for his patience. The library at California State University, Northridge allowed me access to international academic journals that broadened my perspective immensely. And thanks to Sabrina Siskind, who has helped me every inch of the way.

About the Author

J. M. Balakrishnan has graduate degrees in speech communication, speech pathology, and law. She is a national award-winning public speaker and debater. She has served as San Francisco State University's public speaking coach and has taught speech and debate through the University of California's Extension Program, and at San Francisco State University, Pennsylvania State University, and Diablo Valley College. She has also been a debate coach for Piedmont High School and Berkeley High School in the San Francisco Bay Area.

Ms. Balakrishnan holds an MS in communicative disorders and an American Speech and Hearing Association Certificate of Clinical Competence (CCC), and is licensed by the state of California as a speech and language pathologist. After working with over two thousand students in the public school system, she created the Yoga for Stuttering program to help people who stutter. She presently maintains a private practice in the San Francisco Bay Area.